Table of Contents:

We would like to acknowledge **Cardiovascular and Interventional Radiological Society of Europe (CIRSE)** for their invaluable work in advancing interventional radiology education. We also extend our gratitude to **Dr. Mihir Rao and IR Juniors** for their contributions and support in shaping this educational initiative.

Dottir Interventional Radiology Handbook is part of a teaching programme for medical students and resident doctors who want to learn more about interventional radiology. We aim to teach you the CIRSE Interventional Radiology curriculum for medical students and more.

PERIPHERAL ARTERIAL DISEASE

Simply put, **Peripheral Arterial Disease (PAD)** is atherosclerosis of the arteries in the extremities. Risk factors are smoking, hypertension, high cholesterol, diabetes, age, male sex and connective tissue disorders.

It presents as calf pain on exercise known as intermittent claudication, but can progress to pain at rest. If this continues for ≥ 2 weeks it is called critical limb ischaemia (CLI).

DIAGNOSIS

MANAGEMENT

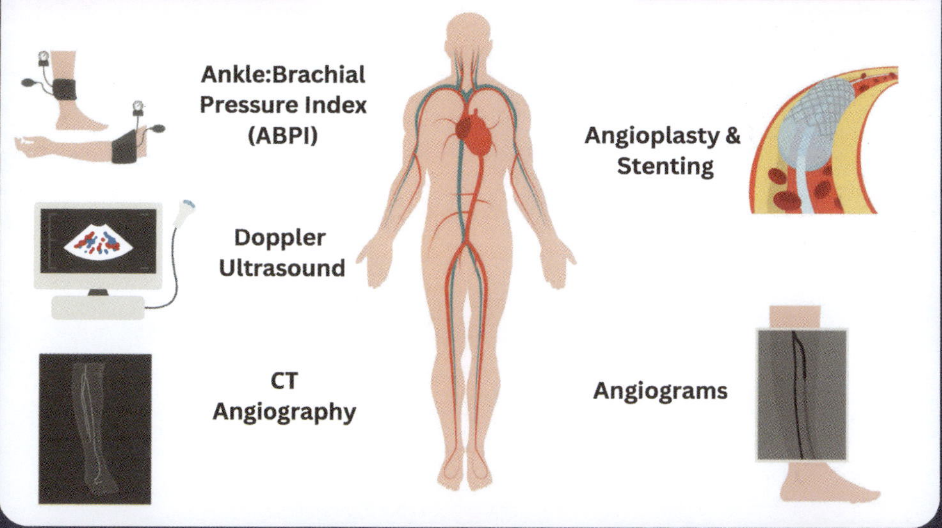

The two classification systems for peripheral arterial disease are Fontaine and Rutherford. Fontaine classifies based on clinical symptoms. Rutherford highlights the different treatments for each presentation. Tissue loss and gangrene are the final category for both.

Notes

ANEURYSM

An **Aneurysm** is a dilation of an artery >50% greater than normal diameter. Abdominal Aortic Aneurysm (AAA) are the most common. Screening begins at age 65 for all men in UK. Along with male sex, smoking and increasing age are known risk factors. AAA can be examined as an expansile, pulsatile mass.

True aneurysms involve all 3 layers of the blood vessel, and false/pseudo aneurysms which arise due to trauma or infection.

DIAGNOSIS

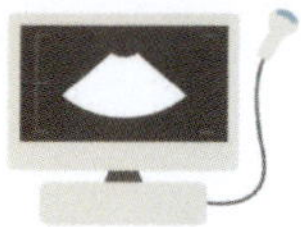

Ultrasound

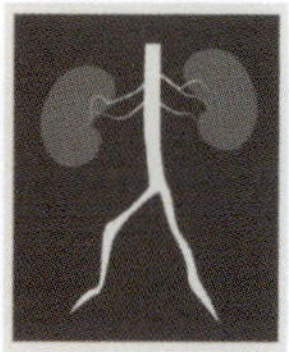

CT angiogram

Incidental finding or AAA screening

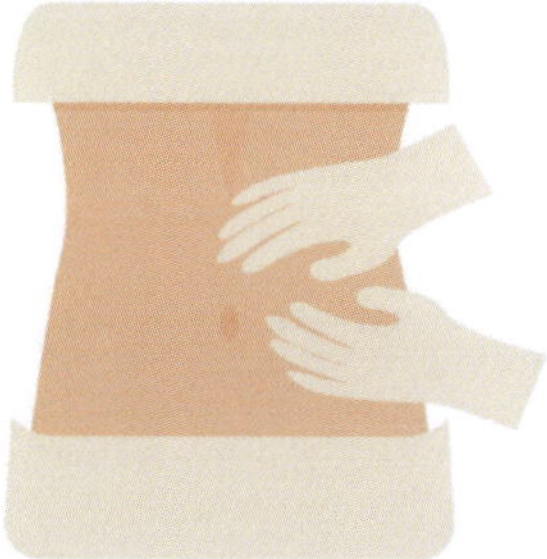

Procedure planning and device selection

MANAGEMENT

Endovascular aneurysm repair (EVAR)
with stent grafts

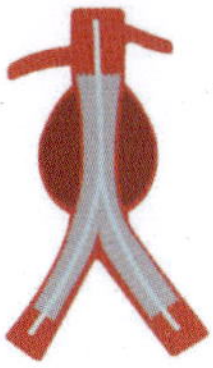

AAA Complications
Aneurysm rupture
80-90% mortality of pre-hospital AAA rupture

EVAR endoleak -
surveillance CT angiogram at 1, 6 and 12 months

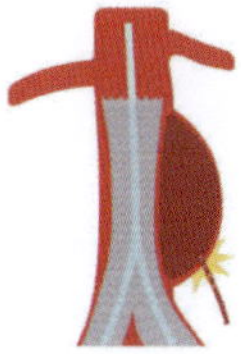

UK AAA Screening Programme - Men aged 65+
No aneurysm <3 cm
Small aneurysm 3-4.4 cm - Annual screening
Medium aneurysm 4.5-5.4 cm - 3 monthly screening
Large aneaurysm >5.5 cm - EVAR or open surgical repair

Dottir
IR Exchange

Notes

Dottir
IR Exchange

VENOUS DISEASE

Venous thromboembolism (VTE) is caused by disruption to Virchow's triad: 1. Sluggish blood flow 2. Vessel injury and 3. Hypercoagulability. Venous blood clots cause deep vein thrombosis (DVT) and pulmonary embolism (PE).

Anticoagulation is the main treatment, but for treatment resistant clots an inferior vena cava (IVC) filter can be inserted. Mechanical thrombolysis or thrombectomy can be used for chronic or extensive clots in veins insufficiently re-canalised by pharmacological blood thinners.

DIAGNOSIS

MANAGEMENT

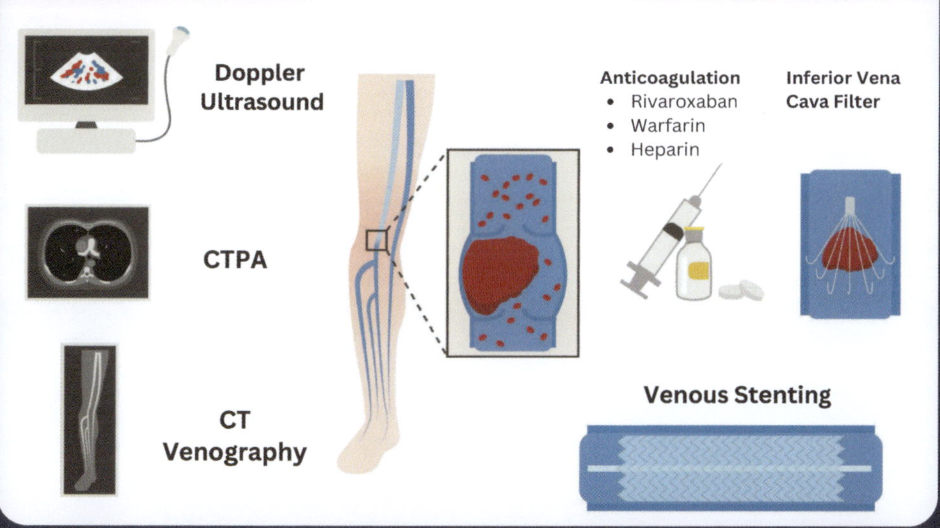

Chronic venous obstruction may occur after venous thrombosis with insufficient recanalisation. This can be due to anatomical venous variants or mechanic/external compression of the vein (e.g. tumour, May-Thurner Syndrome)

Dottir
IR Exchange

Notes

UTERINE FIBROID EMBOLISATION

Uterine fibroids are benign smooth muscle tumours of the uterus. They are more commonly seen in women who are older and of Afro-Caribbean ethnicity.

Patients often present with heavy periods, abdominal pain and pressure symptoms (impacting urinary/bowel function).

DIAGNOSIS

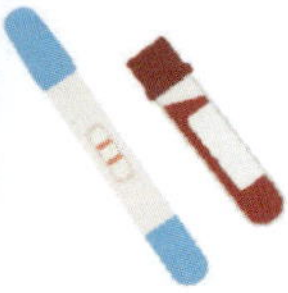

Pregnancy test in women of child-bearing age
Full blood count + iron studies

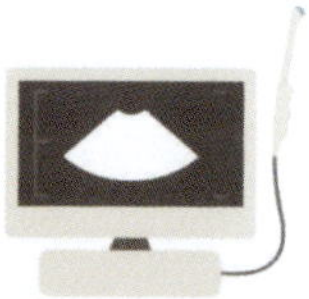

Pelvic ultrasound

Magentic Resonance Imaging (MRI)

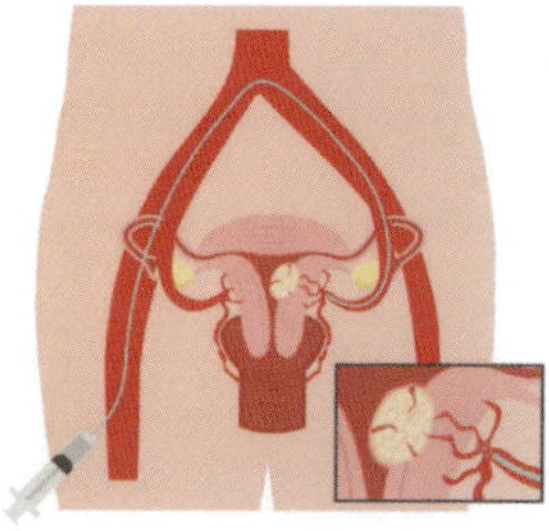

MANAGEMENT

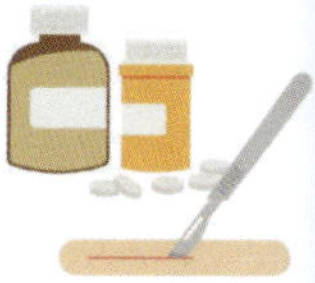

Medical
Mirena coil
Tranexamic acid
Oral contraceptive
Hormonal agents

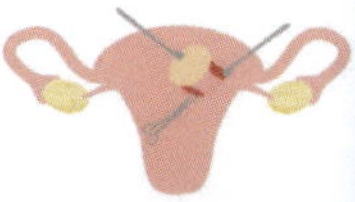

Surgical
Myomectomy
Hysterectomy

IR
Uterine Artery Embolisation with particles

Magnetic Resonance Imaging (MRI) is the best modality for determining size, vascularity and location of fibroids. MR Angiography (MRA) can assess potential collaterals mainly in the ovarian arteries. MRI sequences with different tissue weighting helps radiologists identify red degeneration or non-degenerate fibroids and rule out adenomyosis, adnexal masses, endometriosis and leiomyosarcomas.

Dottir
IR Exchange

Notes

Dottir
IR Exchange

PROSTATE ARTERY EMBOLISATION

Enlarged prostate or benign prostatic hyperplasia (BPH) can cause lower urinary tract symptoms (LUTS): urinary frequency and nocturia. Prostate artery embolisation (PAE) is an effective outpatient procedure for BPH performed in IR under local anaesthetic.

There are alternative surgical options performed like transurethral resection of prostate (TURP). Embolisation has a lower peri-operative side-effect profile and a shorter hospital stay and can also be used to embolise in prostatic haemorrhage.

DIAGNOSIS

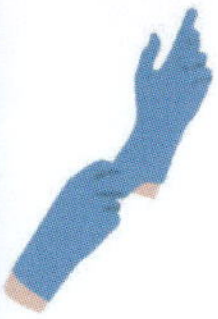

Examination

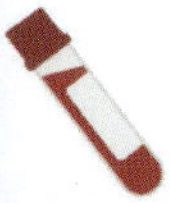

Prostate Specific Antigen Blood Test

MRI

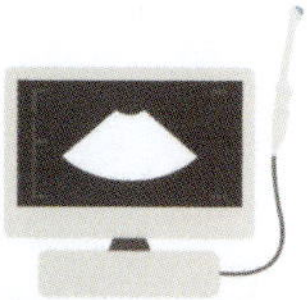

Prostate Ultrasound

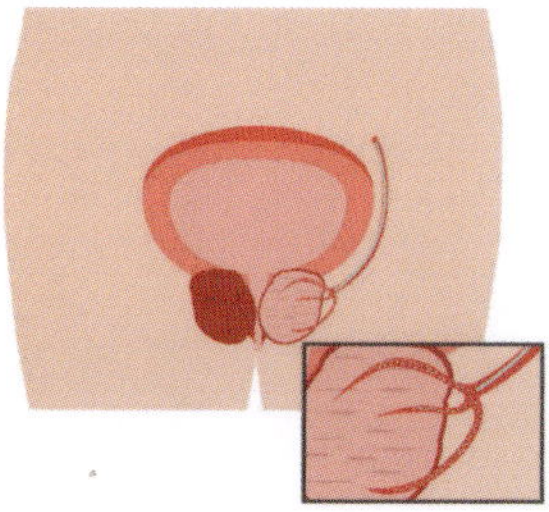

MANAGEMENT

CT or MR Angiography

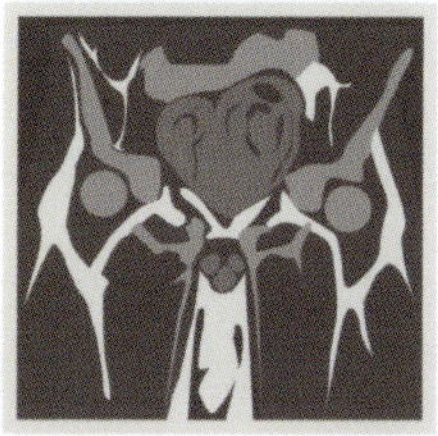

Selective embolisation of prostatic arteries with small particles Gelatin or hydrogel microspheres or Non-spherical polyvinyl alcohol particles

International prostate symptom score (IPSS) for BPH
Eight questions giving a total sympyom severity score out of 35:
0-7 mildly symptomatic
8-19 moderately symptomatic
20-35 severely symptomatic

Notes

GASTROINTESTINAL BLEEDING

Upper gastrointestinal bleeding presents with blood in the vomit (haematemesis) or dark, tarry stools (melaena) due to a bleed from the gut, usually proximal to the Ligament of Treitz.

A lower GI bleed is from anywhere distal to this and presents as fresh red blood in the stool (haematochezia). The bleeding leads to a drop in haemoglobin (Hb) level and a urea rise. Endoscopy is the first-line diagnostic method, but CT angiograms can also detect bleeding >0.3 ml/min.

DIAGNOSIS

MANAGEMENT

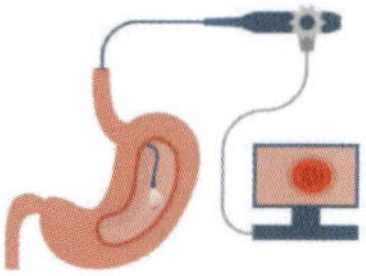

Endoscopy
Oesophagogastroduodenoscopy
Flexible Sigmoidoscopy
Colonoscopy

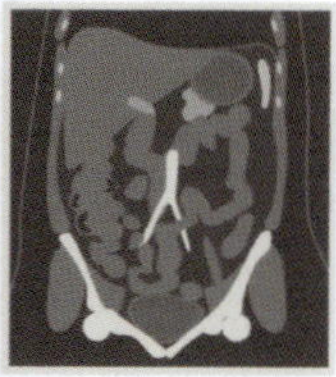

CT Angio
Blood in bowel lumen and contrast exravasation

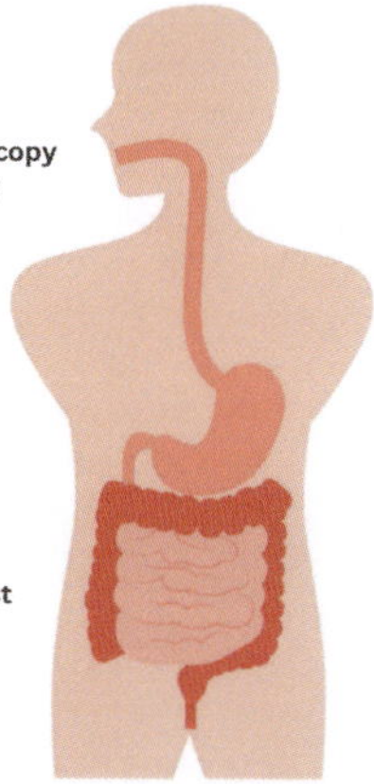

Embolisation

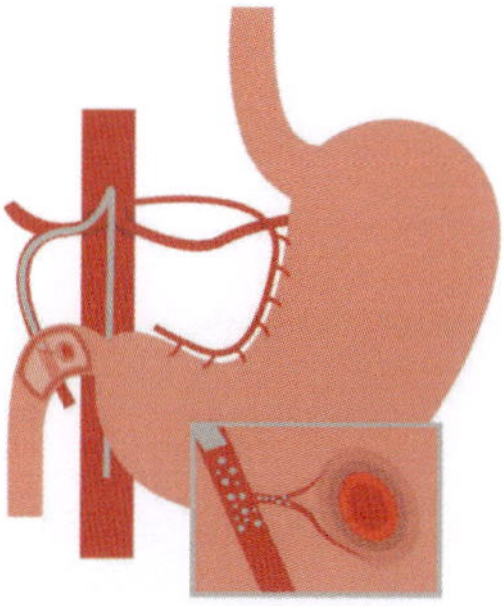

CT Angiography detects bleeding rates ›0.3 ml/min as visible afocal hyperdensities on the arterial phase or pooling of contrast agent on the portal venous phase. Embolisation can performed with a temporary gelatine sponge or permanent coils or glue.

Dottir
IR Exchange

Notes

Dottir
IR Exchange

RENAL DIALYSIS VASCULAR ACCESS

Central venous access is indicated for haemodialysis in renal failure, administration of irritative medications (chemotherapy, parental nutrition) or inadequate peripheral venous access. Dialysis shunts/arteriovenous fistulae are created between the radial artery and cephalic vein with ultrasound guidance.

Types of central venous access: tunnelled catheters and ports, peripherally inserted central catheters (PICCs) and shunts.

DIAGNOSIS

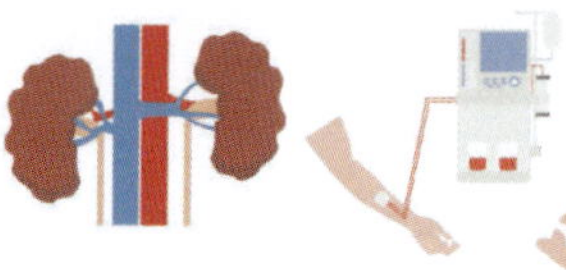

Stage 5 (end-stage) renal failure eGFR <15ml/min

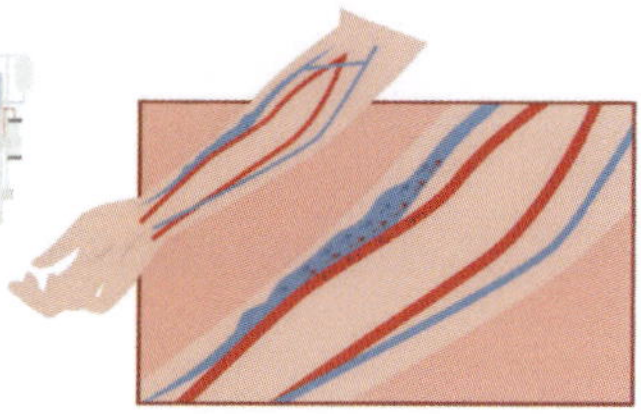

Fistula Formation

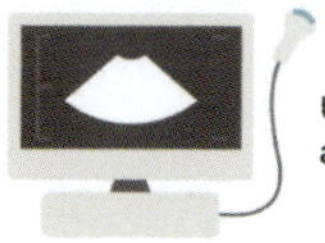

Ultrasound to assess veins

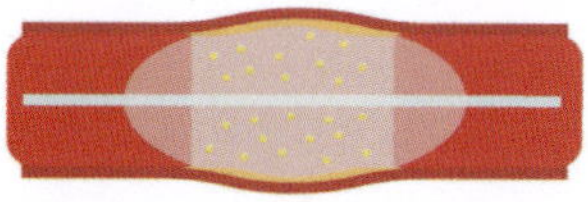

Angioplasty with drug-eluting balloon

MANAGEMENT

Central Venous access

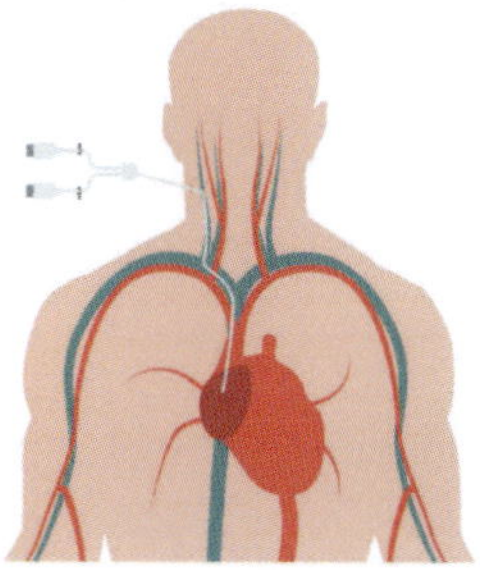

It is now possible to create shunts (arteriovenous fistulae) endovascularly! Blocked shunts can also be treated endovascularly to reopen them with Percutaneous Transluminal Angioplasty (PTA) using drug-eluting balloons ± stenting or stent-grafts.

Notes

Dottir
IR Exchange

BIOPSIES, DRAINAGE & BILIARY INTERVENTIONS

Biopsy: is the sampling tissue or cells for pathology analysis to find aetiology of a lesion to inform treatment; Cytology (Fine Needle Aspiration), Histology (Core Biopsy), Microbiology, Culture and Sensitivity testing.

Drainage: Management of infected fluid collections (empyema/abscess) or mechanical complaints (ascites/pleural effusions);

Biliary Interventions: Patients present with jaundice or biliary sepsis due to obstruction from stones, strictures or stenosis (benign/malignant) which require diagnostic imaging or intervention.

DIAGNOSIS

MANAGEMENT

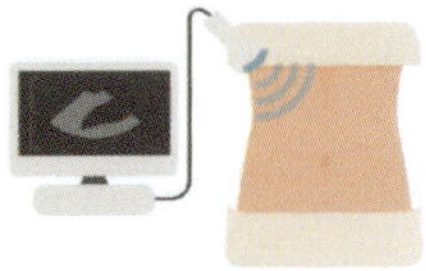

Ultrasound

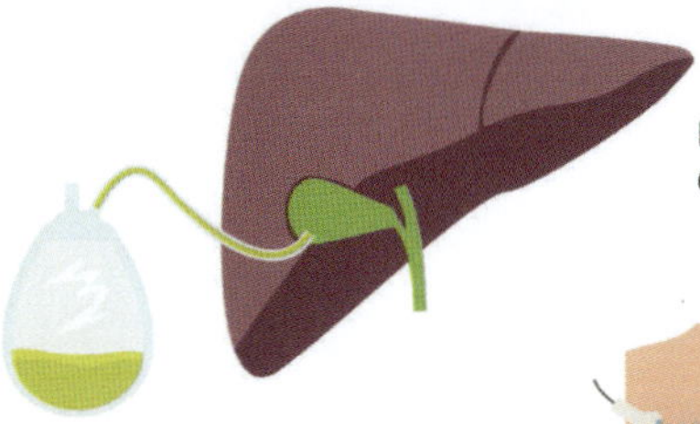

Percutaneous Transhepatic Cholecystostomy Drain

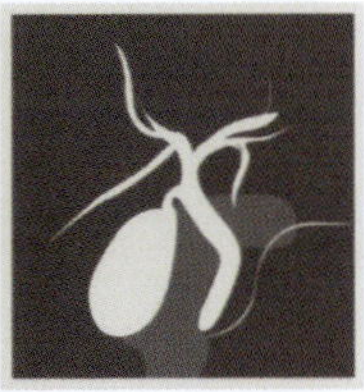

Magnetic Resonance Cholangiopancreatography (MRCP) for imaging biliary obstruction

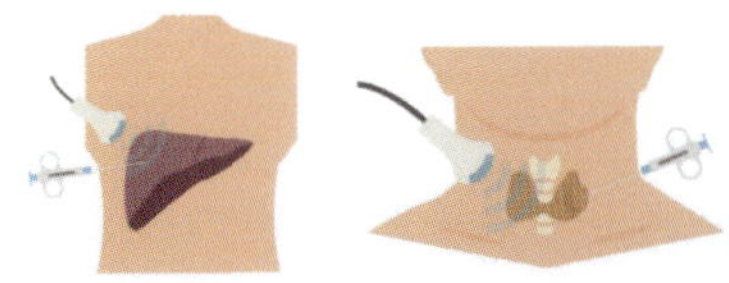

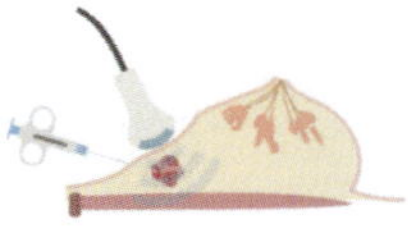

Ultrasound-Guided Liver, Thyroid and Breast Biopsies

Endoscopic Retrograde Cholangiopancreatography is an endoscopic procedure performed by gastroenterology physicians where the common bile duct can be accessed retrograde via the Ampulla of Vater in the second part of the duodenum.

Notes

GENITOURINARY INTERVENTIONS

Obstruction of the ureters can occur due to a variety of reasons including stones, tumours & fibrosis. The increased back pressure from the accumulation of urine can lead to hydronephrosis and impaired renal function.

A **nephrostomy** can relieve this pressure in an infected, obstructed system. Nephrostomies are also be used in managing urinary tract leakage from ureteric damage after abdominal trauma or iatrogenic injury.

DIAGNOSIS

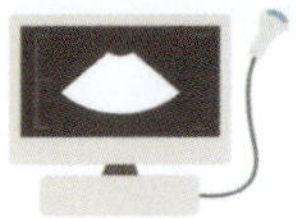

Ultrasound scan

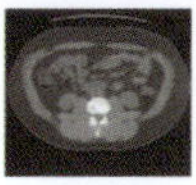

Unenhanced Prone CT Kidneys Ureters Bladder

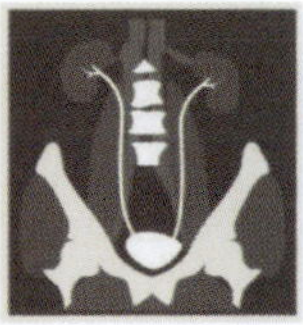

CT urogram
Helps determine cause of obstruction + can help to assess need for ureteric stent

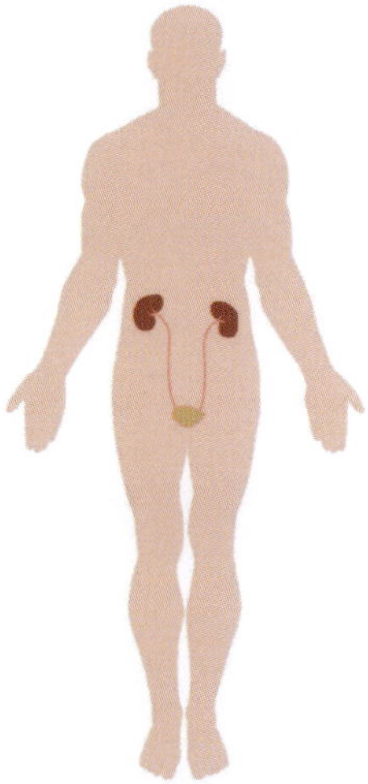

MANAGEMENT

Percutaneous nephrostomy is a procedure in which a thin plastic tube is inserted through the skin to drain urine from the kidney into an external bag.

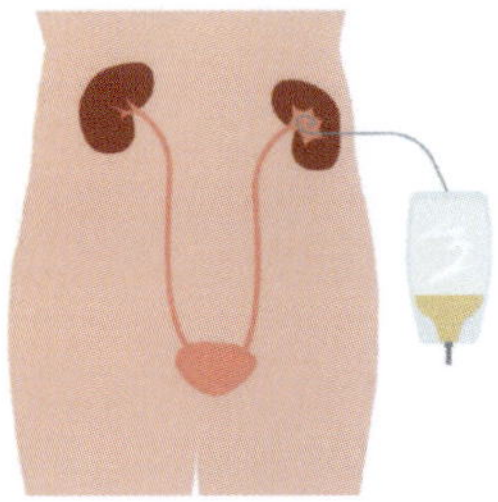

There is a risk of significant bleeding leading to retroperitoneal haemorrhage following a nephrostomy, and close observations for 24-48 hours after the intervention with post-procedure blood tests can help identify such complications early.

Dottir
IR Exchange

Notes

Dottir
IR Exchange

INTERVENTIONAL ONCOLOGY
LUNG & RENAL ABLATION

Tumour Ablation is the direct application of chemical or energy-based (i.e. thermal and non-thermal) treatments to cause local tumour destruction.

Renal Masses are usually incidental findings on routine imaging and are often asymptomatic but can cause back pain and haematuria.

Primary Lung Cancer or metastases are usually asymptomatic early on but can cause cough, haemoptysis, pneumonia and weight loss.

DIAGNOSIS

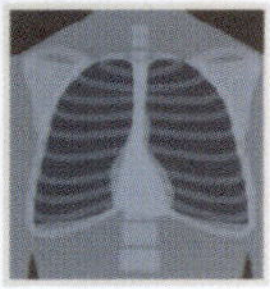

Chest Xray
Main screening tool for lung cancer

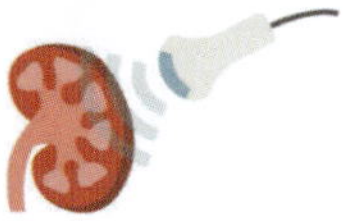

Ultrasound

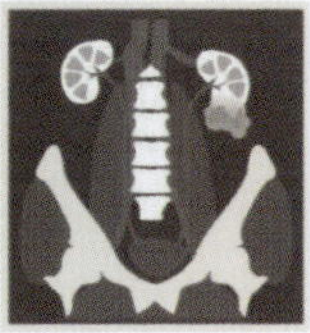

Left Renal Cell Carcinoma Multiphase CT
Helps determine if a mass is malignant, show lymphadenopathy and staging will show lung nodules not visible on plain film

MANAGEMENT

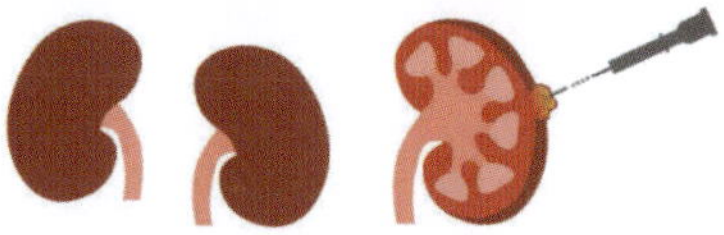

Renal ablation
Poor surgical candidates or small renal tumours
Hot radiofrequency (RF) or microwave (MW)
Cold cryotherapy with an ice ball visible on CT/MRI

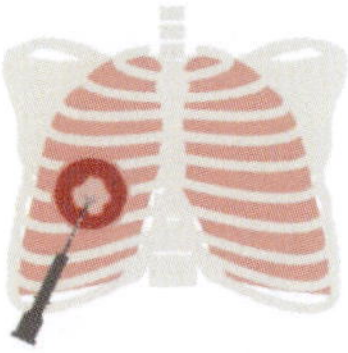

Lung ablation
Primary tumours or metastases
Small (≤3 cm) or few (<5)
Hot RF or MW ablation

Post-ablation CT is performed within a few days to confirm adequate ablation of the targeted lesions and to identify complications such as bleeding, urinary leak, pneumothorax, pleural effusion or abscess formation.

Notes

INTERVENTIONAL ONCOLOGY
LIVER ABLATION & EMBOLISATION

Tumour ablation is the direct application of thermal or chemical treatments to cause local tumour destruction.

Embolisation is the endovascular delivery of particles to deliver treatment, block or diminish blood flow.

Liver tumours can present as jaundice or abnormal liver function blood tests (LFTs) and are usually imaged with ultrasound, CT or MRI. Hepatocellular carcinoma (HCC) is the most common primary liver lesion. Colorectal cancer metastases are the most common secondary liver lesion.

DIAGNOSIS

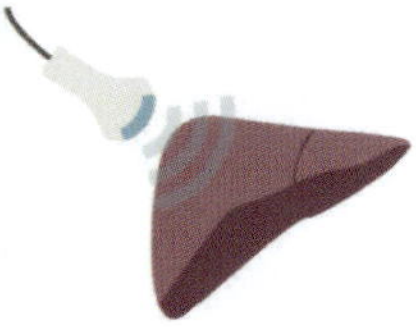

Ultrasound
Main screening tool

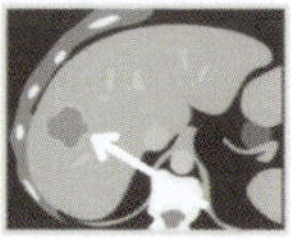

Staging CT/MRI
Helps determine the size, location and type of tumour and plan access for ablation/embolisation

MANAGEMENT

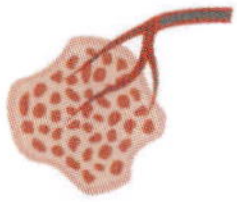

Transarterial Embolisation
(microparticles)

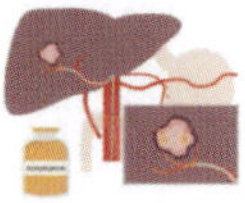

Transarterial Chemoembolisation
(chemotherapy loaded particles)

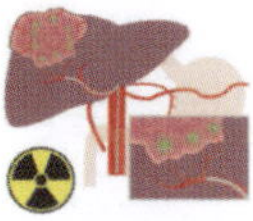

Transarterial Radioembolisation
(Yttrium-90 microspheres)

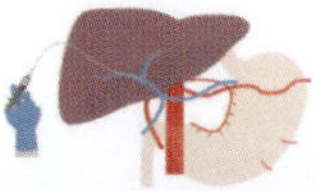

Portal Vein Embolisation
prior to partial hepatectomy to increase blood supply and size of remaining half of liver

Barcelona Clinic Liver Cancer (BCLC) staging A-D and treatment algorithm can help decide which treatment is appropriate

A – Local ablation, Transplant/Resection C – Systemic treatment
B – TACE/TARE D – Best supportive care

Notes

MUSCULOSKELETAL INTERVENTIONS

Vertebral compression fractures can be osteoporotic, malignant or iatrogenic e.g. secondary to steroids, chemotherapy or hormones.

If chronic and unhealed, they cause pain and this is known as Kummel's disease. Fractures due to trauma can be grouped by Magerl's classification into 3 groups. Other differentials for lower back pain include disc tears, herniation, facet joint disease, spinal canal stenosis.

DIAGNOSIS

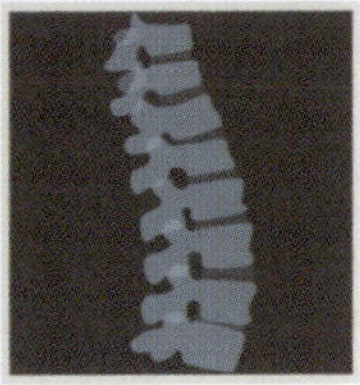

X-RAY

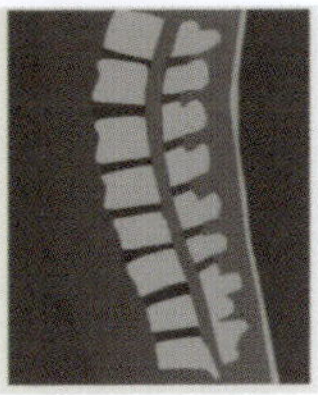

Lumbar MRI
Gold standard for diagnosis of lower back pain

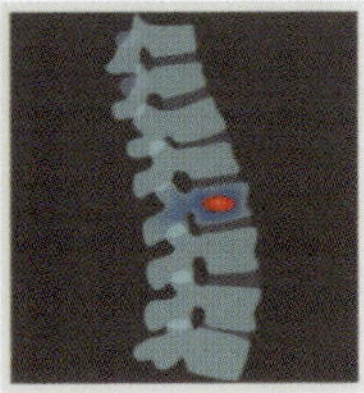

Nuclear Medicine (SPECT CT)

MANAGEMENT

Vertebral Augmentation

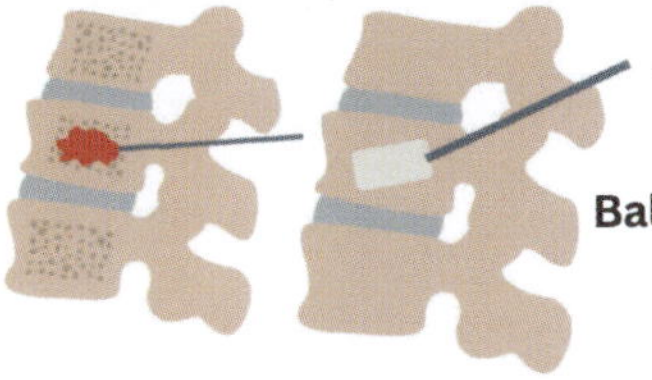

Vertebroplasty:
(Using Cement) = Radiation Therapy if malignant

Kyphoplasty / Stentoplasty:
(Height Restoration)

SPINAL INJECTIONS

(CT/FLUOROSCOPY GUIDED)
ANAESTHETICS/LONG-ACTING STEROIDS

FOCAL THERMOCOAGULATION

FOR FACET JOINTS

Magerl Classification of traumatic vertebral compression fractures
A 1–3 Compression
B 1–3 Distraction
C 1–3 Rotation

Dottir
IR Exchange

Notes

References:

Cardiovascular and Interventional Radiological Society of Europe. CIRSE Interventional Radiology Curriculum for Medical Students. CIRSE, 2024. https://www.cirse.org/wpcontent/uploads/2024/09/cirse_IRcurriculum_medical_students_2024_web.pdf

Dottir
IR Exchange

Dottir

IR Exchange

Dottir

IR Exchange

Printed in Dunstable, United Kingdom

91230527R00018